Tantric Secrets For Men

First Revised-Edition

Kali Bliss

Daka Rocco

http://www.KaliBliss.com

http://www.KaliBliss.com

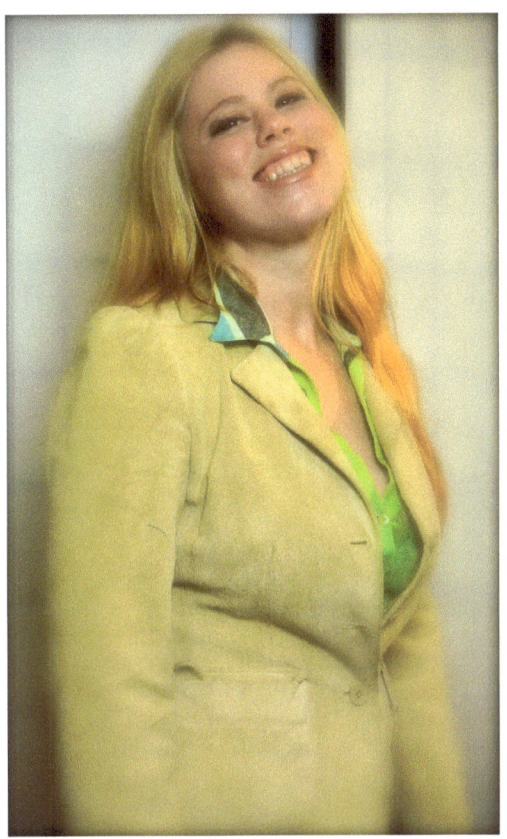

You have started smart by choosing Daka Rocco and Kali Bliss as your guides to Tantra. Kali is an avid sex liberationist, helping people remember the Art of Being Human. Inspired by savoring many varied flavors—as comes with living fully embodied—Kali's motto is "teaching people how to suck the juice out of each moment."

Kali has been a student and teacher of sexual development since she received her bachelors degree in Human Sexuality. Kali also holds an M.S. in Traditional Chinese Medicine and is currently pursuing her PhD in Human Sexuality.

Daka Rocco is an old Tantra Master living his life the way he wants to.

http://www.KaliBliss.com

Learn

How To Use Tantra To Awaken Your Mind
How To Have Long Lasting Sex
How To Use Tantra Sex To Help End Erectile Dysfunction
How To Use Tantra To Help End Excessive Masturbation
How To Use Tantra To Help End Performance Anxiety
How To Use Tantra Sex To Help End Premature Ejaculation
How To Use Tantra To Awaken Your Body

"This is one of the best tantra books, if not the best tantra books I have ever read. It is oriented specifically towards men. Guiding you step-by-step on your erotic, spiritual journey. The step-by-step is amazing. This is the first time I have ever been able to have multiple orgasms! I recommend this for everyone!" -Robert Chase The Arizona Dating Guru

"This book changed my life. Not only did it improve my sex life but it taught me to have much more self confidence with the opposite sex. It is like Kali knew what I was thinking when she wrote this book. I wouldn't miss reading it for the world. I will continue to re-read it as needed." -Dustin S. Seattle, Washington

Dustin suffered from 7 years of erectile dysfunction.

There is a lot of really sound, powerful information here. The problem some people may have is that they won't get it without being given the same information five or six times. There is no filler, just master keys for male sexuality. The best thing about this book is that it really made me want to learn more. If a book can do that while providing really good content, it gets my recommendation."

-John Michaels author of "Survival In Any Situation: Build Your Ultimate Go-

Bag."

People are raving about this new development in Tantra… What has prevented you making this sexual transformation up until now is behind you. This first edition of Tantric Secrets For Men is on how-to harness the power of your sexual energy to help prevent and put an end to all problems brushed under the sheets.

At the end of this book you will learn more about…

"SECRETS to Magnetizing Your Sexual Senses!!!

How-To-Instantly Change Your Energy-Vibrancy To Get What You Want In Bed… (Even if it's considered socially unacceptable, fun and exciting)… In 3 Days Or Less! By Using The Advanced Tantra-For-Men-Oceans of Sex-Process™

…Without Any of The "good-goody" B.S!"

WELCOME… If you desire to acquire a knowledge of the GREAT SEXUAL AWAKENING that has dawned upon mankind with the birth of the twenty-first century—with a mind and heart open to those scientific and spiritual truths that are daily being proven by scientists and thinkers of world-repute—we take the liberty of reminding you there is no program more enlightening, no work more appreciated, no effort more powerful, than this first revised-edition of Tantric Secrets For Men.

There is a difference between this program and others upon the subject—it is not an ordinary chronicle of unconnected notations but a romantic story of extraordinary interest and value for the sexually spiritual and scientific truths which set forth the most advanced knowledge of the deeper things of the Soul so simply that any reader of ordinary intelligence can grasp, comprehend and apply those laws whose values extend the usefulness of every Truth seeker who is seeking light upon the MYSTERIES OF SEXUAL ENERGY IN THIS LIFE, both Here and Hereafter.

Women commonly joke about how two intense desires rule and govern men and control all of your thoughts, your joys and sorrows. They are your two appetites, a hunger for delicious food and the craving for sexual passion. Curiously enough, while our society takes great pains in educating us to make a salary and prepare to gratify the gustatory hunger, the much tabooed question of sex has been excluded, in our present civilization, from every discussion.

Yet sex lies at the foundation of society, it permeates unconsciously the thoughts, aspirations and hopes of humankind. Sex and raw passion is glorified as the source of the most admirable productions of art, of the sublime creations of poetry and music; it is accepted as the mightiest factor in the masculine building of civilization, as the basis of the family and state. The ego of power and the passion of sex are self absorbing in all the positive ways once could be. Even though we are told these acts of power and sex are wrong, that we have to be moral!

Morality is basically a set of very general rules concerning what to do and what not to do, generally involving large consequences. Blindly using someone else's moral code, tends to reduce your competence, because it prevents the forming of proper cognitive links between actions and consequences. To be free you need to formulate your own moral code.

In its right appreciation, sex has been exalted by the ancients in song and story and extolled by priest and philosopher. "To the Spirit, to Heaven, to the Sun, to the Moon, to Earth, to Night, to the Day, and to the Father of all that is and will be, to Eros." Such an invocation was possible only among the ancient civilized nations. They recognized the importance of the sexuality to life. They could not see any moral guilt in actions of lust. Sex was regarded by them to be a design of nature and as pure success.

They discovered passion to be the focus of life. For this reason sexuality among the ancients was an object of pure reverence as the fundamental force of life. The divine adoration of sex was the practice of every tribe and nation of prehistoric antiquity. Even the organs of sex were considered intensely beautiful and pleasurable objects, and were treasured. The lingam, the Sanskrit term for the male sex-organ, and the yoni, the external female genitals, were symbols of the worship of the ancients and were objects of special religious rites.

Before Christianity, the worship of reproduction was the dominant religion known to mankind. Sex-worship was not confined to any one race. It was the form of worship common to all primeval nations of the globe. The rites of passage, placed the lingam in such high-esteem that if the potency of a practitioner were to deteriorate the entire village would mourn. Ancient texts explain how men up until their 90s were meant to have sex every day for rejuvenation. Now we find ourselves in the Millennium and with technological advancements most of the population pops pills when we have sexual problems or give up sex at a very young age instead of taking the time necessary to worship sexual health.

The aim of "Tantric Secrets For Men" is to get you back to the root of you true nature as a man-to worship pleasure and the health of your loins.

Understand all of us should be incredibly sexual. Having sex with as many women and men as we desire but because of strict morality we find ourselves prevented by shame and guilt to explore the biological drive to procreate with many to spread the fruit of our loins. What gets in our way? Negative beliefs and emotion, they distort our ability to perceive pleasure.

How you perceive pleasure is characterized by the senses. The development of the senses is key to great spiritual sex. When the six senses: sight, sound, touch, smell, taste, & proprioceptives become heightened with the techniques in this book you will experience life-changing pleasure.

When we loosen up to be guided by our senses and desires and needs, we then can find freedom within ourselves, to enjoy our bodies and heighten pleasure.

Within us is a subtle energy, an energy which has been clearly outlined in the ancient Taoist texts. Tantric sexual practices allow us to have a direct experience of that energy. You can harness the power of each sexual energy, and there are several, and direct it's flow. You will feel and sense this energy.

Imagine those times when you felt a magnetic pull between you and a prospective lover. Whatever label you give this experience, it is entirely pure energy. An embodied reality of pleasure that flows along the meridians. Many Tantric practitioners report that their lives enter a higher stage of development after they experience this energy.

With this book you will be able to tap into the power and direct the flow of sexual energy to have longer lasting sex, to help end premature ejaculation, to help end erectile dysfunction and other ailments that cripple the masculine divine.

The side effects of Tantra for men can be bigger and better orgasms although; we create freedom from being orgasm driven. Orgasm for many becomes a means to an end. The pleasure from the orgasm is often isolated into the genitals for these people.

In Tantric Sex, we use the energy from the orgasm to have a spiritual experience similar to Savikalpa, where the body is in a trancelike state, but our consciousness is fully perceptive of its blissful experience within. The exterior world fades off into the distance and so do our beliefs that no longer serve us. When we allow Savikalpa, to enhance and orgasmic like state that will ripple from head-to-toe for many hours.

When you are in an trance-like aroused state, the Tantra practitioner uses 'Eccentration' a form of peripheral vision. 'Eccentration' is where you gaze into the distance with no fixed-point on which to focus. You will then become visually aware of the sexual energies arising from the human body in the focal plane. The feeling of time passing is stretched with 'eccentration.' There is a revelation that time, a distinct quasi-physical dimension in itself, is not the same as the feeling of time, a product of the senses. You will experience this shifting of time when doing the master keys listed in this book.

The Science Behind Sexual Energy

Sexual energy can be found when taking a deeper look into the meridian system.

Meridians are like copper traces on an electronic circuit board, running throughout the body. They act as pathways of positive and negative energy power, which communicates to the various body parts including the lingam. Western physicians believe these meridians interrelate with the nerve pathways. The nervous system is comprised of neurons and fiber, when triggered it creates feelings, movement and emotion within a particular body part. The nerves also dominate the ability for muscles to contract and relax. Lets think back to orgasm and how you feel during orgasm.

Orgasm is the sudden discharge of accumulated sexual tension resulting in rhythmic muscular contraction characterized by an intense sensation of pleasure.

The intensity of the sensation depends on how the energy concentrates and moves down the meridians which, hyperlinks with the nerves.

If a person is experiencing low quality erections without it being a side effect from diabetes or coronary disease, this could be because the energies have become irregular.

What do I mean by irregular energies?

The flow of energy in the meridians can become irregular in many ways. This can include deeper or slower than normal flow, reversed flow, or altered electromagnetic charge.

If you go to http://www.TantraResources.com I will show you in a video how to energy-test and correct the balance of sexual energy running through your system.

When energies are irregular they can have an effect on how you maintain an erection. In a recent study done by the John Hopkins University School of Medicine in August of 2012, they found that there is a feedback loop in the penile nerves that trigger waves of nitric oxide to keep the penis erect. Within the penile nerve tissue the nitric oxide is produced. If the person is experiencing irregular energies it is my finding that it diffuses the nerves from producing the chemical reaction necessary to maintain an erection. This is why it is so important to know if your energies are running correctly.

Imagine there is a river but, it has rained for weeks and dams are forming. What happens to how the water flows? One area of the river will dry up and another area of the river will overflow. If we were to use the dam metaphor for what happens when premature ejaculation and when erectile dysfunction occurs it would be...

Erectile dysfunction occurs when a disturbance in the system prevents the energy from flowing to the nerves to create nitric oxide in the penile tissue to form in order to maintain an erection.

Have you ever seen erectile dysfunction? Even with visual sight, laymen can tell no energy is moving through the lingam. The lingam appears to be flaccid, lackluster in color and cold in temperature with erectile dysfunction. Often this is accompanied with bouts of performance anxiety. Unfortunately the anxiety causes the release of adrenaline from the adrenal gland that acts to constrict the blood vessels, including those that lead to the penis. A vicious mind-body cycle is often created that turns anxiety into potency problems.

 In the upcoming chapters you will learn how to calm the mind with Tantra and direct sexual energy to the lingam to get and maintain erections easily at any age.

Premature ejaculation occurs when a disturbance in the systems swells with an abundance of energy to the nerves, which results in excessive pleasure you can no longer control. In Chinese Medicine the etiology is called 'kidney Qi not firm.' This means pleasure floods the boundaries creating an unsustainable flow of energy within the meridian.

Through these chapters you will go back to your natural state as a man. You will learn how to harness the power of sexual energy. Allow the techniques you are about to learn to give you freedom from being orgasm driven as you experience more full body pleasure and more control over your ejaculation.

How To Awaken Your Body

Every man dwells in a world made up of external reality and of its own sensations. Much of the complexity of human existence is due to this double aspect of life.

We perceive the external world in which we dwell and have our physical being in the first place through the instrumentality of our senses. Touch is the sense which yields the earliest information concerning the realm of sexual existence which extends beyond the sentient body.

It is the most diffuse of the senses. Every portion of the bodily surface is sensitive to contact though particular regions are especially sensitive. The primal touch sense is also differentiated into a number of special sensations. Throughout all sentient existence touch retains its character of directness and immediacy—and generates the most intense feeling of "being alive." This is the sense we are developing when we awaken the body.

Touch is the sense that awakens the dormant energies. You are probably familiar with the concept of Kundalini, a very dormant energy, or maybe you're not so allow me to explain.

Through meditation and engaging the correct sexual energy flow through the following techniques listed later on in this book, the Kundalini is awakened, and can rise up from the muladhara chakra (root chakra) through the Chong Mai internal and external pathways also known as Sushumna in Kundalini Yoga. The internal pathway of Chong Mai runs into the Mingmen, the 'Furnace of the Gate of Life' which to many when activated feels like a full body orgasm mutilating their contextual reality.

If you think about the symbology of Kundalini: she is presented as a snake wrapped three and half times around a smoky grey lingam. Imagine if a serpent were to awaken from a slumber, do you think it would be kind to you? It would be hungry, irritable and wanting to stretch its limbs. It is said, Shakti when aroused will bring you back to source if you like it or not.

Once you have experienced Kundalini, you must remember to bring yourself back down to reenter contextual reality. I use a special type of metal coin on the muladhara to close the energy centers. Edgar Cayce, the world-renowned health psychic of the 20th century, originally advised for the metal coin. He explained it grounded the muladhara because it brought the user back into contextual reality. I keep a coin on me at all times. If you do not have a coin it is like you are a walking target for the muladhara to soak up negative energy.

A long time student of mine started making the coins after he had a near death experience. He was hit by a boat while swimming at Lake Powell in Arizona and was left dead for several minutes. Ever since then he hasn't been the same but, this special metal coin makes him cognizant of his physical body otherwise he'd be floating off into the ethers unaware of contextual reality. You can get the coin on my website http://www.TantraResources.com/products it is only available for a limited of time.

There are many ways to intensify Kundalini arising in the body by using Chong Mai to lead into different levels of awakening. We will use the sense of touch to connect up the energy in this upcoming drill.

Master Key: Kundalini Awakening Drill For Men

These are not quick fixes but serious methods that will take time. You can get this drill on video and audio by going to my website.

Make sure that the room temperature is warm, preferably around 78 degrees Fahrenheit. Find a comfortable place. Sit with your back straight. It's important that you are not lying down or slouching as you might fall sleep. Make sure you won't be disturbed by closing the door and turning off or placing the phone in silent mode.

Close your eyes and press your eyelids. The pressure you should use is the same as pressing your eyelids without any discomfort. Always use your fingertips.

This practice is done alone. First start with the process of Nalinaksha, breathe in deeply through your nose and out through your mouth (time—15 to 20 seconds).

1. Place the middle finger of one hand on the Ajna (between your eyebrows above the bridge of your nose-third eye).

2. Place the middle finger of the other hand in your navel.

3. Gently press each finger into your skin, pull it upward, and hold for 12-30 minutes. Often a spontaneous sigh or deep breath signals that the energies have connected over from central meridian to governing meridian.

Nalinaksha

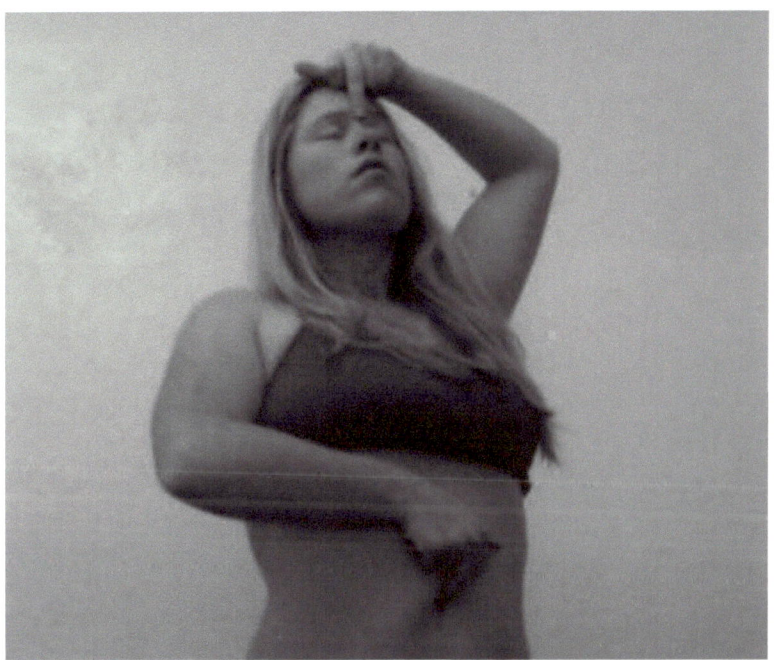

After Nalinaksha you will go into the touch-filled erotic meditation of Shiva Bruitao. Some Tantra Masters believe Shiva Bruitao is the alchemical process of distilling seminal fluid and diverting it to the brain.

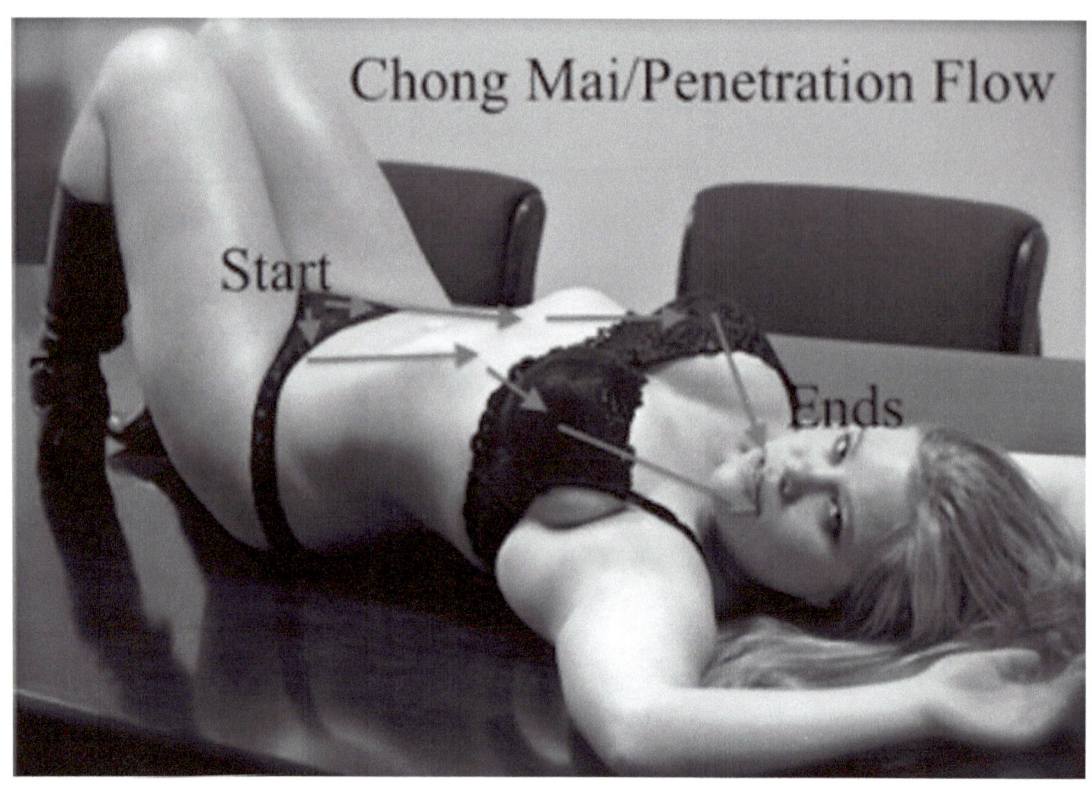

Shiva Bruitao

Become familiar with the sexual energy flow of Chong Mai in the image with Kali Bliss. This is one of the pathways used to stimulate Kundalini awakening. Although orgasms characteristically result from genital stimulation, there are many accounts suggesting that non-genital stimuli from Shiva Bruitao also generate feelings that have been described by men as orgasms.

1. Begin the meditation by locating the perineum; this is the space between your anus sphincter and testicles.

If you are familiar with Mula Bandha, also known as Root Lock in Ashtanga yoga, this advanced Tantra For Men drill will be very easy for you.

2. Breathe in through your nose and as you exhale through your mouth engage the pelvic floor, drawing it upwards towards your navel. If you don't know how to access the pelvic floor, imagine a space between the pubic bone and the tailbone.

*If you are new to this, you may need to contract and hold the muscles around the anus and genitals, but really what you want is to isolate and draw up the perineum, which is between the anus and genitals.

When I'm first working with a client on this exercise, with non-toxic markers we color this area on their body. I then sit them in front of a mirror; have them lift up their scrotum so they can visually see the upward movement as they contract the pubococcygeus muscle. This creates a powerful synesthesia, coupling three of the senses together: sight, touch and proprioception.

The perineum is the location where two dominant sexual energies, central meridian and governing meridian meet in the body with Chong Mai.

3. As you imagine the energy isolated in the perineum as a bright white light. It is now concentrated since the contraction sealed off any energy leaks. You can direct the energy with your intention.

The key to intention is turning off internal dialog, the voice that runs in your head, you can do this by placing the tip of your relaxed tongue on the back of your front teeth. Then shut your mouth. Put your right hand over your frontal neurovasculars and breath in through your nose and out through your mouth until you feel the pulses on your forehead.

http://www.KaliBliss.com

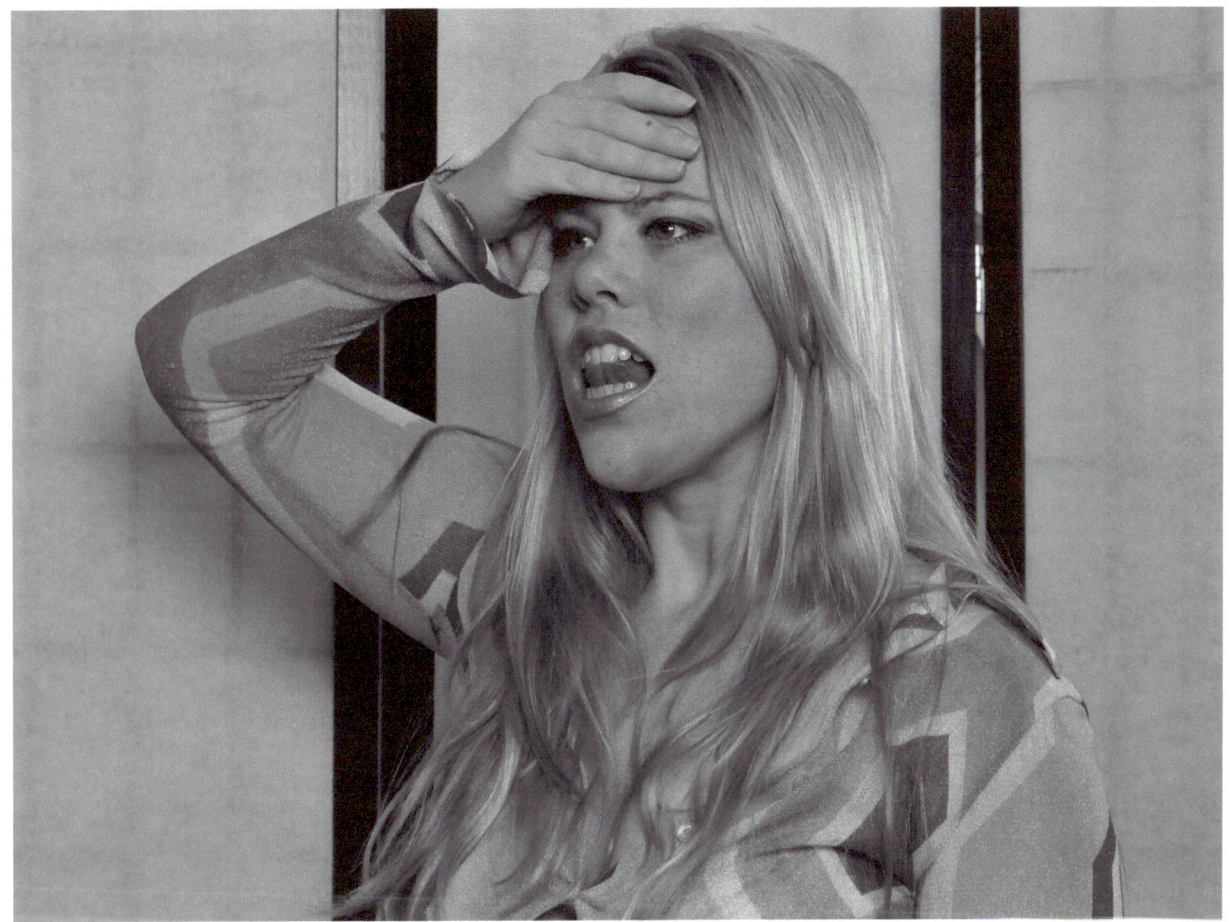

4. Once you feel relaxed and the internal dialog is shut off, trace slowly up the midline of your lingam with your left middle finger as if barely touching it.

5. Imagine a beautiful naked lover that can fulfill your every wish. Gaze upon the lover as if they are there in the room with you. Imagine it is their hand streaming softly up the midline of your lingam.

6. As you feel the first surge of arousal, give it a color, the color red, and pulse the color red and the feeling of arousal up your Chong Mai by using your left middle finger to trace up from the perineum and encircle the lips.

7. Work yourself up into a sexual fantasy while still maintaining the Mula Bandha and repeating upward traces of the Chong Mai every time you feel surges of arousal.

*When you get close to orgasm, trace Chong Mai backwards from lips to perineum until the ejaculate is reabsorbed and the erection retracts into a flaccid state. Then with the right hand trace 1 time the correct flow of Chong Mai from perineum to lips.

I know the master keys of Shiva Bruitao can be confusing. If you go to website I will show how to do this in a video http://www.TantraResources.com

Benefits of Shiva Bruitao:

-Orgasm without ejaculation

-Awakens the body through tactile sensation

-Engages Kundalini awakening

http://www.KaliBliss.com

-Dormant energies like Chong Mai create more pleasure

Please understand Shiva Bruitao is an advanced Tantra method for men who have practiced for many years the lineage of Sjhain. I know this book will make waves in the Tantra community since these secrets they don't want the general public to know. If you see any negative comments under this book on Amazon you will now know why. There are many competitors out there that feel this information you should not have.

How To Have Long Lasting Sex

To focus on lasting longer, we really need to look at a bigger perspective. So that would involve seeing that sexual energy is our life force energy.

Sex is not just a stress release thing, when we have sex with our lover there is a much bigger exchange going on than just the obvious.

There are many components to long lasting sex. The obvious to long lasting sex include the high pitch of constant arousal, the essentials of foreplay and of course, sexual positions. When those three components are met, we then include an advanced master key in Tantra. This is the ability to go deep into a sexual trance-like state, meditating on how energy moves through the meridians. When this is done, you will create more intense pleasure for what seems to be hours.

The first meridian we will meditate on is the kidney meridian. You can learn more about this meditation by going to my website to view the video.

The kidney meridian is regarded as the body's most important reservoir of essential energy. The original prenatal energy (*yuan qi*) which, forms the basis of life is stored in the kidney organ-energy system, which is why the kidneys are also known as the 'Root of Life.'

From my time studying sexual energy in Chinese Medicine School, we learned the kidney organ system also includes the adrenal glands. The adrenal sit like hats on top of the kidneys and secrete a wide range of hormones that trigger emotional states, including anxiety. Another reason why it is so important to keep this sexual energy flow in top health is to calm the mind during sex.

The kidney meridian also includes what ancient Chinese Medicine call the 'external kidneys:' known as the testicles in men. The kidney meridian is thought to control sexual and reproductive functions and provide the body's prime source of sexual vigor.

The start of the kidney meridian at K-1 (The Well Spring of Life Point).

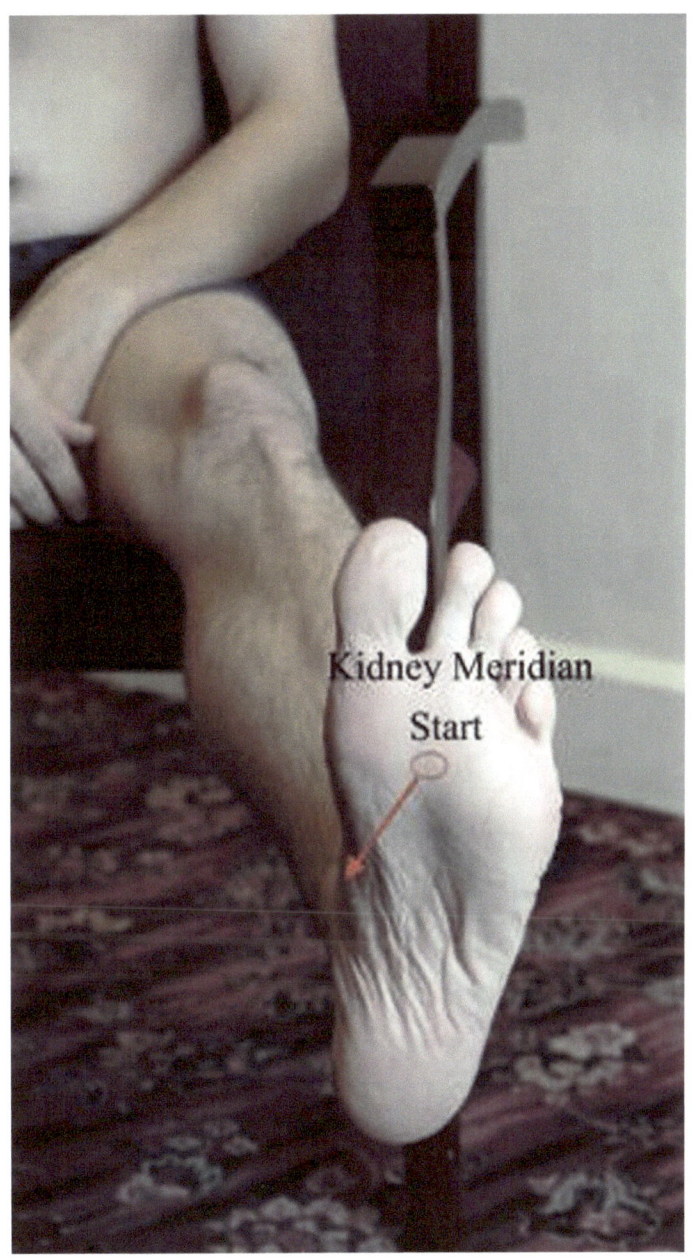

Kidney Meridian

Start

The kidney meridian continued. The end point below the clavicle located at K-27.

This meridian directly affects the intensity of sensation felt through the lingam.

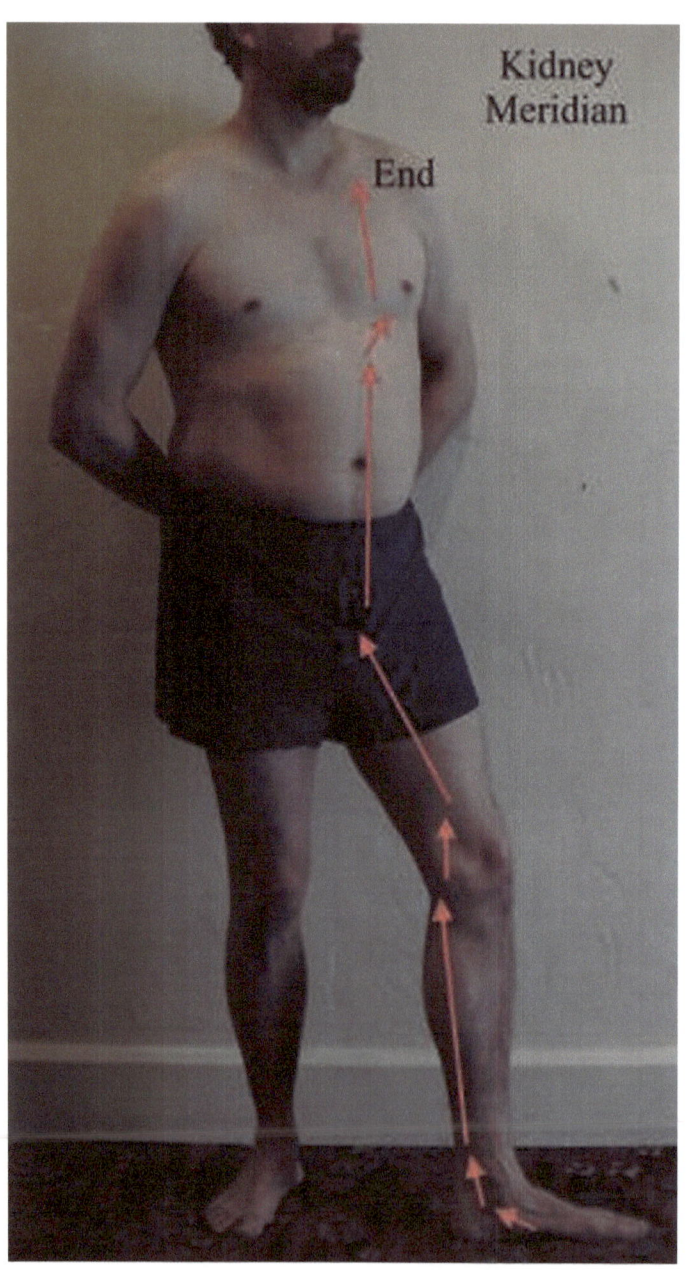

When you get aroused do you tense your calves? This is a direct result of primordial sexual energy flowing up from Kidney 1 and into the calves as the energy makes it way to the lingam and up to the ending point at Kidney 27 just underneath the clavicle.

Master Key: Kidney Meridian Activation Drill For Long Lasting Sex

When sex doesn't last long, this means often times our senses have merged into one. This is where you'd want to hyper-focus on just one sense indirectly related to tactile pleasure. Out of the sixth senses, the primary sense dissociated from the kinesthetic-tactile is the olfactory sense. In this drill, we will be working with the olfactory (smell) and the tactile built-in sense of releasing tension in our calves during orgasm that is directly related to the kidney meridian. From now on whenever you come close to orgasm your sense of smell redirects the sexual imagination.

There is much about the qualities of odors that appeals to the imagination. Odors are inconstant, irregular, apparently immaterial, vague, yet penetrating. On certain occasions they intoxicate the mind.

Odors lend themselves to curious personal idiosyncrasies, on account of the intimate associations they are capable of invoking. Immersed as we live in a world of odor, the associations roused by the sense of smell contain endless possibilities. It has been said, smell is the essence of the soul.

German author, Patrick Suskind, wrote a book called "Das Parfum," about a man born with no body scent who begins to stalk and murder virgins in search of the "perfect scent." It is one of my favorite literary novels since it depicts how the sense of smell can carry an emotional meaning. This is why I prefer to pick scents that carry seductive influence, like the smell of your lover's hair or the smell of their yoni dripping with beads of pleasure.

1. Trace the kidney meridian three times from the beginning-to-ending points before coitus. Breathe in through your nose and out through your mouth imagine Shiva coming down from the heavens above you to engage the powerful Vajra.

2. Go back into the physiology of sex. Perhaps you are on the bottom and the woman is on top of you. Lye on your back, completely naked and imagine a beautiful woman is on top of you gyrating her hips and you are about to orgasm.

3. Tense your calves, lift up your hips and all of a sudden imagine the smell of mud. As you smell the mud, notice how there is now a sensation of walking through mud on the balls of your feet (this activates Kidney 1 to open up instead of tightening with sexual energy).

4. Instantly replay this scenario over in your mind 100 times real fast as if on fast forward.

5. Imagine a time in the future when, if it had happened in the past, you might have been tempted to orgasm, and tell me what you do instead.

You have just invoked the control, discernment and passion held so tight between Shiva's thighs. Envelope into the tidal wave of his power; become one.

Sensual Drills For Long Lasting Sex

We represent the world using the visual (images), auditory (sounds), kinesthetic (touch and internal feelings), gustatory (tastes) and olfactory (smells) senses. We picture ourselves lying on a bed, hear the voice of your lover moaning, feel the sensation only a warm mouth on your lingam can produce, taste the sweetness of your lovers lips and smell the aroma of her shampoo wafting into your nostrils.

Our thinking consists of these images, sounds, feelings and usually for some, tastes and smells. The entirety of our experiences has been recreated through these senses in our memories and governs our capabilities and beliefs about sex. This is why it is so important to enhance the quality of the movies we live inside of our minds by doing the following sensual enhancement exercises.

Visual

Stand in front of a mirror naked while you do the following.

     1. Start by seeing your skin tone

     2. Notice the curves of your body

     3. See your face flushing

4. Watch your penis grow erect in a mirror and notice the stages.

Kinesthetic

Sit down on the bed naked. Close your eyes while you touch yourself. Be very slow and relax your mind.

1. Touch your skin from your inner thigh to the top of your hand, under your fingers

2. Touch the hair around your testicles

3. Feel the tips of your toes being licked

4. Touch the base of your penis

5. Touch the tip of your penis

6. Touch behind your knee

7. Feel the cool air on your steaming hot body after you release an orgasm

Auditory

Close your eyes and remember hearing these experiences.

1. Hear the sound of your hand and lingam make as you masturbate

2. Remember the voice of a lover as she moaned your name

3. Hear the erotic sound of your exhale

4. Hear your heartbeat race faster and faster when you get closer to orgasm.

Olfactory

Close your eyes and remember these aromas.

1. Smell your lover's hair

2. Smell the scent of you ejaculate

3.   Smell the sweat during sex

Gustatory

Close your eyes and remember these tastes.

1. Taste the sweetness of your lover's lips

2. Taste your lover's yoni

3. Taste a large ripe strawberry

4. Taste and feel the texture of your lover's nipples

Which sense provided you with the most vivid experience? Which was the weakest? Once you figure this out, it is then easier to control how you experience the reality around you by focusing directly on the sense to either enhance it or decrease it.

Lets say you are a high visual with no staying power when it comes to sex. You would want to focus on enhancing the other senses during sex by paying attention to them. Example: you are sucking on breasts. The breasts are in your face and they really turning you on. You notice the texture, the salty taste and take account for how she is processing in the moment. I explain more about sensory dominance and sex in a video if you go to http://www.TantraResources.com

How To Help End Erectile Dysfunction

According to the Journal of the American Medical Association, in 2011 more than 105 million Americans have reported struggling with chronic erectile dysfunction and many of them were not aware that there is natural help for them.

Only those who suffer from erectile dysfunction know how difficult and annoying it can be and what a great hindrance it causes in one's sex life. These problems don't allow a couple to take the full pleasure and advantage of physical intimacy and with the passage of time; it can lead to deep conjugal dissatisfaction. This is why it is so important to find intimacy without having goal-oriented orgasms. Although ejaculation does move stagnant fluid, which has ripened in the testes; it is important to release. Imagine stagnant water on a warm stove.

Ejaculation is something you have to continuously exercise; once you stop the hormones decrease. The ancient Taoist believed that sexual activity was a natural process until the day you died and reincarnated. This was taken from the book 'Classic of the Simple Girl' (Sui dynasty 581-618), it gives an indication of the recommended frequency of ejaculation for men according to their age and condition of health. Of course, this should not be taken literally, but only as a theory.

Frequency of Ejaculation

20s	30s	40s	50s	60s	70s
2x/Day Healthy Once/Day Declined Health	Once/Day Healthy Every Other Day Declined Health	3 Days Healthy 4 Days Declined Health	5 Days Healthy 10 Days Declined Health	10 Days Healthy 20 Days Declined Health	30 Days Healthy None Declined Health

The Taoist treatment for Erectile Dysfunction takes into account releasing the stagnant energy ripened in the testicles. Allow me to explain the depth of Kidney Qi relationship with your erections.

The Kidney-Essence is the organic basis for the transformation of Kidney-Yin into Kidney-Qi by the warming and evaporating action of Kidney-Yang. The Yang aspect of Kidney sits in the point that most acupuncturists refer to as the Mingmen (the mingmen is located between the two kidneys)–the furnace that ignites the raw sexual energy to spread throughout the body.

Kidney-Yin and Kidney-Yang have the same root and they rely on each other for their existence. Kidney-Yin provides the semen and Kidney-Yang heats the penis into an erection. They are fundamentally one and interdependent, deficiency of one necessarily implies deficiency of the other, though always in differing proportions.

Think of an oil lamp. Kidney-Yin is the oil, and the flame is Kidney-Yang. If there is a reduction in the oil (Yin), the flame (Yang) will reduce; if there is an intense increase in oil (Yin) the flame (Yang) will get smothered.

The state of your sex drive [I like to call "essence"] determines the state of the Kidneys. If Essence is flourishing and abundant, the Kidneys are strong and there will be great vitality, sexual power and fertility.

If Essence is weak, the Kidneys are weak and there will be lack of vigor, infertility or sexual vulnerability. Aging itself is due to the physiological decline of Essence.

When the mind has been stressed, when the body has been sexless, when you feel undesired, the Kidney Qi has become stagnant. The energy of the semen has to release even if it is not in the fluid form of ejaculate.

To do this, I like to use secret acupuncture points that only few acupuncturist know about. You never have to needle these points, you can hold them with your middle fingers for the same effect. Finger pressure varies with the physique. If you're over weight, you are more likely to experience tenderness and in that case, gradually apply pressure.

Light pressure should be taken into account:

-This is your first time!

-Swelling in the genitals!

-High blood pressure!

-Heart trouble!

Hard pressure should be taken into account:

-Chronic pattern of erectile dysfunction!

-If your pain tolerance is high!

Press against the point of the skin surface, in a small circular movement, about 2 or 3 cycles per second. Start bilaterally on the points, for an example: Kidney-1 to Liver-1 on the yang side (right side of the body) then work over to the left side of the body (the yin side).

This is to create a smooth flow of vibratory energy throughout the body by stimulating various organs, glands and cells that are interrelated to sexual arousal.

The period of treatment can range from one minute to five minutes for each set of points per treatment, once a day, or whenever you have the problem, or whenever you feel you wish to do it.

A yawn can mean the release of stagnant energy, or even flatulence or burping can indicate such. If this happens, breathe deeply and release.

Caution: Keep your hands clean, and nails should be trimmed to prevent injury. Avoid working on open wounds, scars or bruises. If your erection lasts longer than four hours please consult a physician

Points to hold to remove stagnant Qi inside of the lingam and testicle associated with erectile dysfunction.

Liver 1: Located on the dorsal aspect of the big toe, lateral corner of toenail (inside corner, closest to the heel). Dadun Liver 1 is the Jing-Well Point of the Liver meridian. (image on next page)

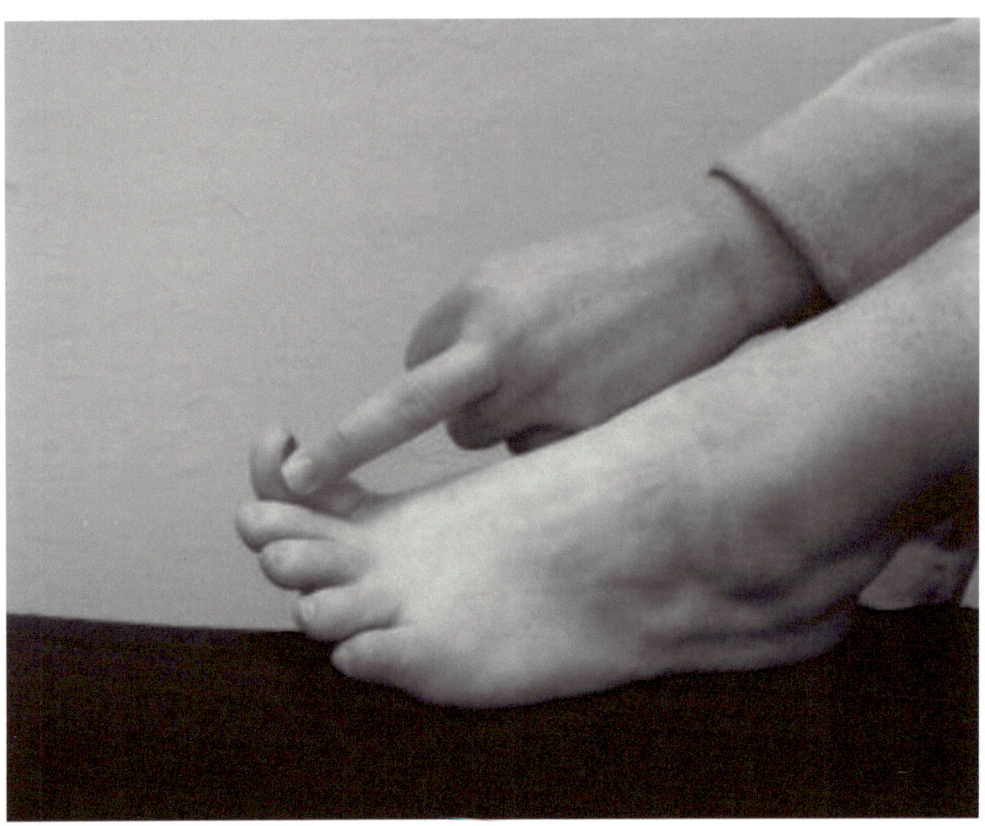

Kidney 1: Located on the **sole of the foot**, between the second and third metatarsal bones, in a depression formed when the toes are curled together.

Hold simultaneously Kidney 1 to Liver 1 for 3 minutes.

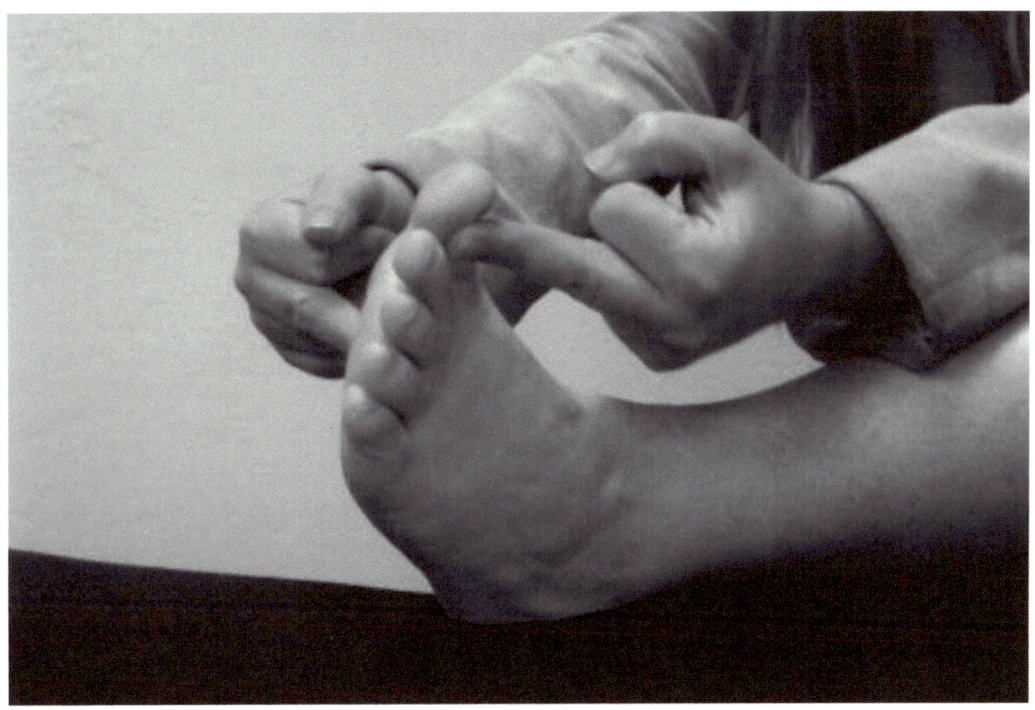

In addition to acupressure treatments, herbs can potentially rebalance the stagnant energy in your lingam. One herb specifically for increasing kidney yang and removing stagnation is called Hu Lu Ba and the other Lu Jiao Shuang is derived from deer antler and is used to strengthen the kidneys and improve kidney yang. Acupressure, herbs and Tantra blend together to form a synergistic approach to erectile dysfunction.

In Tantra, when a man is experiencing erectile dysfunction we bless the lingam with mantra and apply a salve to the lingam. The salve is made from castor oil which is a traditional folk remedy also known to be so powerful it adopted the name the *Palm of Christ*. Castor oil is mentioned in the famous Egyptian medical text, the Ebers Papyrus (written in roughly around 1550 B.C.) on healing sexual ailments and erectile dysfunction.

The Art of Blessing allows the Supreme Energy, which is beyond existence and non-existence, to flow over the person. This helps us to detach from everything that chains us, helps us discover divine wisdom without being affected by the whirl of life, leading us to final liberation. It teaches us that every human function regardless of state, is a divine manifestation, which enables us to more intensively, and more often experience, feelings of love, compassion and forgiveness.

I was inspired by Dr. Masaru Emoto's work, where he taped paper strips on bottles of tap water and then photographed the frozen water. He found that words such as "Thank you," and "I love you," caused the tap water to form beautiful crystals (see picture at left). Words such as "You make me sick," or "You are a fool," caused ugly, distorted crystals or no crystals at all.

When you think about the negative thoughts you have held in mind about your performance imagine how your body responds. Approximately 72 percent of a human body is made up of water, and our sexual organs fill with fluid when we're aroused. Of course, any toxic belief or positive blessing will affect your performance.

When giving a blessing to your Lingam it is important to say, "Thank you." This is done by hyper focusing your mind on each layer of tissue within the lingam.

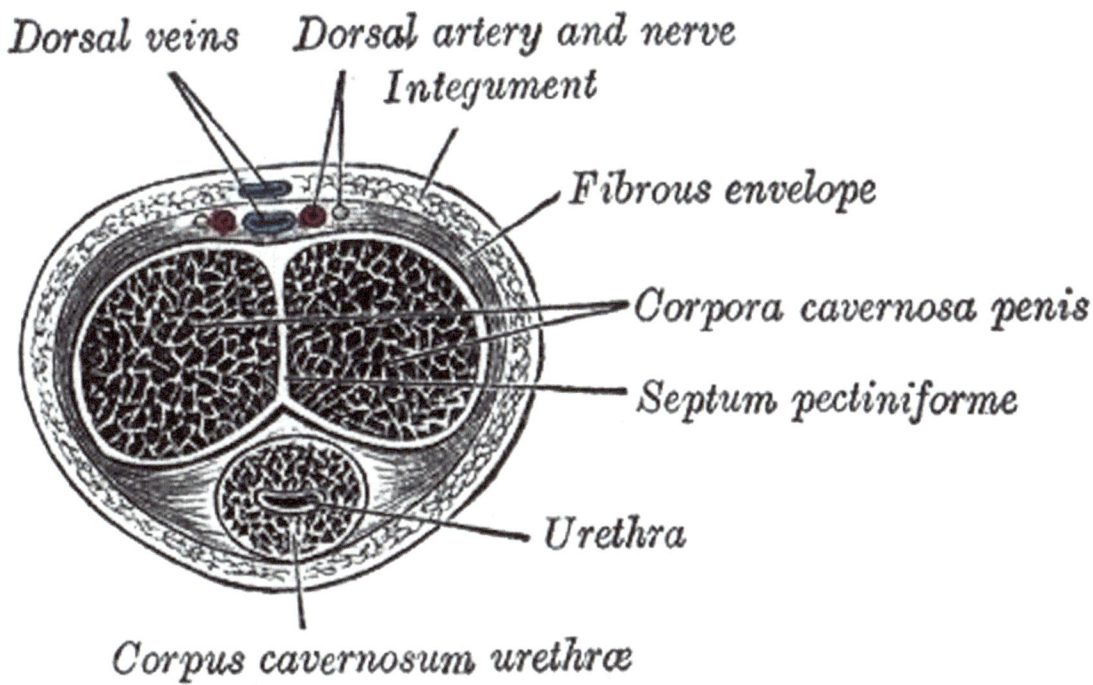

Look at the diagram above then look at your lingam. Close your eyes and imagine going deep into the septum pectiniforme and once you're fully engulfed inside of the tissue and becoming one... [This does take some meditation skills]. Say aloud, "Thank you." This is done to all 7 internal compartments of the lingam.

There is an audio program on my website that takes you deep into a trance-like state to bless the lingam. Once you bless the lingam you'll notice instant change with your performance! http://www.TantraResources.com

How To Help End Delayed Ejaculation/Excessive Masturbation

A man with delayed ejaculation either does not have orgasms at all or cannot have an orgasm until after prolonged intercourse which might last for 30–45 minutes or more.

Frequent masturbation without ejaculation stimulates the parasympathetic nervous functions. Excessive stimulation can result in over production of sex hormones and neurotransmitters such as acetylcholine, dopamine and serotonin.

Abundant and unusually large amount of these hormones and neurotransmitters can cause the brain and adrenal glands to perform excessive dopamine-norepinephrine-epinephrine conversion and turn the brain/body/energy functions to be extremely sensitive. In other words, there is a big change of overall chemistry when one excessively masturbates and cannot ejaculate.

Sexual desire and ejaculation is strongly associated with healthy Kidney energy. If the kidney meridian is weak, in particular if kidney-yang is deficient, there may be a lack of sexual desire. If kidney-yin is deficient leading to a rising empty-heat in the meridian, there may be excessive sexual desire with in an inability to be satisfied with excessive masturbation.

Clearly it is a healthy sexual behavior, and more people should masturbate. The key to having ejaculation while experiencing delayed ejaculation is to stop having sex. Your Kidney Qi is depleted and you must take respite from sex.

You need foods, which calm the nervous system and your mind and help build the fluids of the body. Foods that are helpful are sweet potatoes, squash, potatoes, string beans, lemons, black beans, kidney beans, oysters, clams, duck, and chicken eggs. Especially oysters! Oysters contain dopamine, which increases both sexual desire and testosterone levels. They're also high in zinc, which is necessary for proper sexual function in men and, more importantly, semen production.

How To Help End Performance Anxiety

Male sexual function depends not only on sound physiological health but also on the psychological state. 'Mental restlessness' is a translation of the Chinese expression 'Xin Fan,' which literally means 'the heart feels vexed.' Anxiety and extremes of emotion, which destabilize the Heart and the shen, can also wreck havoc with the ability to achieve and maintain an erection.

Suggested Chinese Herbs:

Tian Wang Bu Xin Dan

Gui Pi Wan

Shi Quan Da Bu Wan

You can find all the herbs on my website http://www.TantraResources.com

Daka Rocco has something personal to say to you right now on how to curb performance anxiety. I have to warn you his letter is filled with all of that fun toilet-Zen. If you can't handle a little dirty humor than don't read his letter.

Dear Friend,

I'm about to share with you several reality principles you must know to get out of performance anxiety state.

Reality Principle #1: You Deserve As Many Erections As You Desire!

"A clever female seducer would announce,

"Let's not make love, let's certainly not fuck at least this time," while putting her arm around your waist and running her fingertips on Viagra-energy points, and licking these erogenous zones with the tip of her tongue. As she repeated that we were not going to have sex, I felt a chill up my spine and my cock harden."

Reality Principle #2: Erections And Orgasms Are Delicious Fun!

By eliminating the pressure, and encouraging the natural "Viagra-Energies" to take root, couples often have a tendency to mature into their sexual abilities. And in achieving erections without pressure, they teach themselves how to have sex that last longer than a sixteen year old jerking off to his peers on Facebook at all hours of the day. If your erection lasts longer than four hours please consult a physician immediately.

Viagra Tao,

1. In search of a lost erection, stop looking! Thoughts like, "Oh my god, wouldn't it be awful if I didn't get it up," is almost guaranteed to keep it soft. Awareness of Murphy's Law ("if something can go wrong, it will") applied to male potency, often creates the problem.

I must, I must, I must—I will—am I—aren't I—I'm not? If the whole time is spent worrying, 'is it gonna work this time?' Then it takes all the fun and spontaneity out of sex.

2.   As your boner subsides, let it. Each man has his own response to a fading erection. If the penis starts getting soft, trying to reverse it with these key Energy Viagra Points will help. Have her work for it by holding the points.

3.   Be where you are. If you find yourself butt naked in an embarrassing situation—well just be there. Hang out with it. Accept it. Don't apologize to yourself or the lady if you are not "producing" or living up to some stallion standard. Be where you are. Who you are.

You've got to be willing to make a fool of yourself in bed. If nothing is happening or you're a two-pump wonder. So what? Go grab a banana off the kitchen table, or you can take a breather!

Reality Principle #3: There is always another boner—boners are plentiful!

Sincerely,

Daka Rocco

Daka Rocco is an initiated Tantra Master. He is one of the few men still living today that holds into account the ancient traditions while using a form of humor called Toilet-Zen.

There are many points to hold for performance anxiety. The images below help quiet the mind and put you into a state of relaxation. Hold simultaneously the point for up to three minutes. This is a light palpation as if you are barely holding them. Done only with the middle fingers and thumb. Kidney 6 to Heart 6.

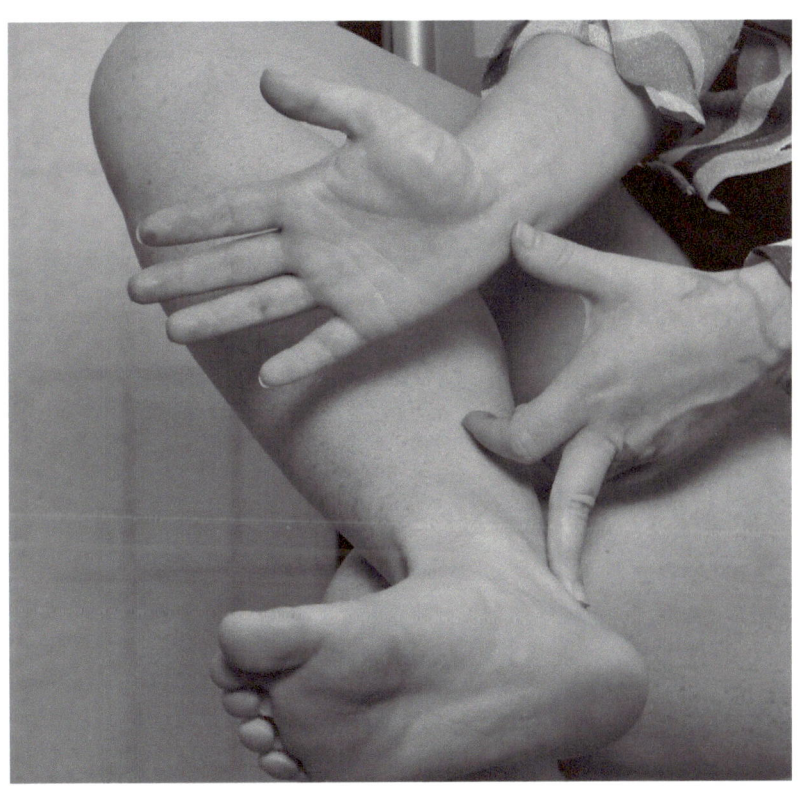

How To Help End Premature Ejaculation

Premature ejaculation is defined as an uncontrolled ejaculation either before or shortly after sexual penetration, with minimal sexual stimulation and before you wish it to happen. In Tantra, to help end premature ejaculation we use our senses to gauge how aroused we have become. Think of the sixth senses and take note of what excites you. Is it the tingling sensation? List everything that excites you on a scale of 1-10. List by order which one excites you the most to the least.

Hold governing meridian 4 to central meridian 4 (image below) with both hands. Breathe in through your nose and out through your mouth as you imagine the excitement releasing through these two points. These two points are known to hold in all of our excitement.

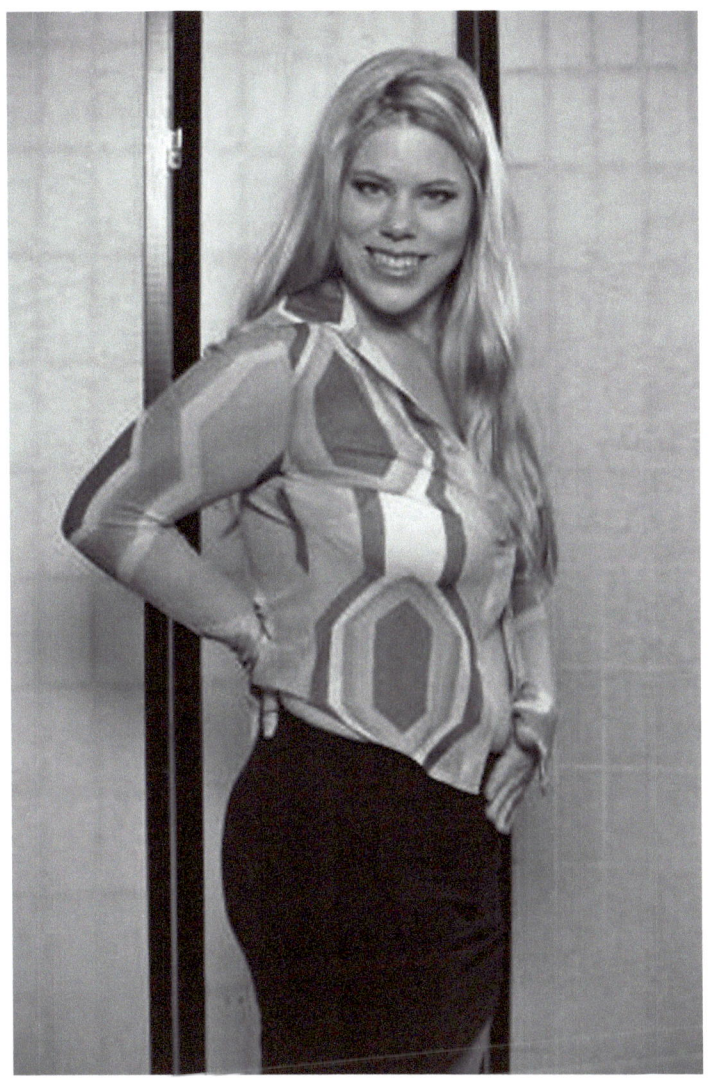

Central Meridian 4 to Governing 4

Conclusion

The one thing to learn and accept about your sexuality as a man... Is how sex is your primary source of nurturing, contact and also how you evaluate yourself in which you feel successful and good as a man. To the extent that a human expression of love as sex is the most powerful experience of divinity that most of us encounter, man looks to the power of his body for that expression whether it be his brains or his hands.

In Tantra, a sexually free man doesn't try to remake the world or his friends or his family. He merely appraises every situation by the simple standard: Is this what I want for myself? If it isn't, he looks elsewhere.

If it is, he relaxes and enjoys it — without the problems most other people take for granted. A sexually free man uses his tremendous power of choice to make a comfortable life for himself. The power of choice. You have it. But you forfeit it when you imagine that a great sex life depends on external attachments like Viagra and people. But you can choose for yourself — from hundreds of exciting, happiness-producing alternatives and do natural preventative processes. The power is within you.

Why not use that power? These are 'Tantric Secrets For Men.' You decide which information you will use or not use.

You decide what your next action will be. You decide what moral code you'll live by…To be sexually free of all the problems brushed under the sheets, you have only to make the decision to be free. Sexual Freedom is waiting for you — anytime you're ready for it!

"SECRETS to <u>Magnetizing</u> <u>Your</u> <u>Sexual</u> <u>Senses</u>!!!

How-To-Instantly Change Your Energy-Vibrancy To Get What You Want In Bed… (Even if it's considered <u>socially unacceptable</u>, <u>fun</u> and <u>exciting</u>)… In 3 Days Or Less! By Using The <u>Advanced</u> <u>Tantra-For-Men-Oceans of Sex-Technologies</u>™

…Without Any of The "good-goody" B.S!"

What do I mean by "good-goody" BS?

It is sort of like the old nusery rhyme, "Girls are made of sugar... and boys are made of slugs and snails." That is just sheeple training done to the masses!!!

I <u>do</u> like The Rolling Stones version much more.... "Am I hard enough?

Am I rough enough? Am I rich enough? I'm not too blind to see…"

I <u>don't</u> like following rules of conformity. I <u>don't</u> like the church telling me the rules of sex. I <u>don't</u> like being considered a slut because I have slept with more than seven people at one given time.

I <u>do</u> LOVE the strong possibilities of living what others call "The Wicked Ways" of non-conformity… Having lots of sex with really powerful people without having to commit…Having all the good things I LIKE…even to being considered the villain by others that fear how others will view them.

I <u>don't</u> like learning Tantra from a Tantra Master that teaches me to "think alike" and be "nice" all the time and does fluffy energy work with just a hand job.

I <u>do</u> LOVE training with a Grand Master that has taught real Tantra orgasmic living and can give you an orgasm with a single touch, and is an extremely humble being. I <u>don't</u> like the government regulating divorce or marriage. I <u>do</u> LOVE doing and getting what fearful people call "The Forbidden Fruits," of sexual peak performance which can helped be achieved in Kali Bliss' Oceans-of-Sex-Technologies™

From: The Desk of 'Jessica Williams'

Date: December 12, 2012

Time: 2:11 PM

Dear Friend,

I'm glad you liked Tantric Secrets For Men. When I walked into the office this morning Kali Bliss was in the same place I had left her at 5PM-tpying madly on her new Mac. I asked her if she slept. She looked at me and said,

"I've learned through life, that when I had feelings (good or bad) and I didn't act on them I was greatly left behind and some could even say, <u>"punished for not acting on them."</u>

And when I had feeling sto "<u>do something</u>" and <u>I acted on those feelings with my intentions,</u> I was greatly rewarded beyond belief."

Those words have stuck with me all day. Have you ever had a time like that? When you were left behind. Up until this point what has held you back from emersing yourself in the possibilies of real Tantra? You read the book, didn't you-otherwise you would not be here learning about the deeper possibilities of your sexual energy.

Maybe you don't believe in energy, maybe you don't believe there is any hope for you. Well, maybe it is time to show some of the powerful things that can happen once you start doing the drills we're about to teach you in this very letter!

Maybe it's time to show you that learning 1 drill... and only 1 drill... can have an overwhelming change in your life. But I wouldn't believe me quite yet.

Before you even start that, I'd like to point out a "Wicked-Mind-Map" I made about how the **Advanced Oceans-of-Sex-Technologies™** has helped some of our private clients in the last 30 days. (Yes, this book was revised in December of 2012 so these **real life studies** happened in November and December of this year!!!)

Let me WARN You!
I am going to include some SEXY-PICTURES in this letter.

*The pictures are for **PROOF ONLY**. Nothing else is intended behind them. Some pictures will show how one of my clients, a skinny geek added massive attractor fields to his root chakra INSTANTLY AFTER he'd implemented advanced oceans-of-sex-technologies™*

The photos have been blurred to protect the identity of the man and most men don't want to gawk at another man's fruits.

So let's begin:

Advanced Oceans-of-Sex-Technologies™ Private Client PROOF STORY #1

"Skinny Geek Turns Sexual Magnet Gets Married To Soul Mate He Only Known For 6 Weeks Who Has High Sex Drive"

I call him a skinny geek because he is 6'4 130 pounds (you do the math) and is a software developer whose hobbies used to include everything BUT girls. He is honestly one of the nicest people in the world with one of the biggest hearts I have ever met.

Let me give you a back story to this Oceans-of-Sex-Technologies™ Client.

Jaime was struggling to meet and keep a girlfriend for the past 11 years. The longest relationship he had up until this point, was in high school that lasted 8 months. Jaime's life-goal has been to find and keep a loving woman, but he couldn't ever do it, because he felt romantically stunted even after going to guru after guru (sound familiar? I hope so, because you got to admit it first!).

From me, this Private client #1 got his hands on Kali's **Oceans-of-Sex-Technologies Training™** and **within literally 42 minutes** literally met a beautiful Asian goddess in a taxi they shared. Within hours they were sharing smiles over food and before this skinny geek believed he was invisible to most good-looking women. After six weeks they happily married!!!

Imagine being able to notice that someone was on the wrong frequency for getting what they want… they wanted to listen to 101.5 and they were on 98.1 frequency. That slight **energy change** was really the difference for him.

Just like Boiling Water. If you're at 99.9 degrees Celsius the water will NOT boil. But when you change the dial 1/10th of a degree to the right, and "WALA" you have Boiling Water. It's the same with Oceans-of-Sex™!!!

Here is one of the photos of him and his wife. I cropped their faces to protect their identity.

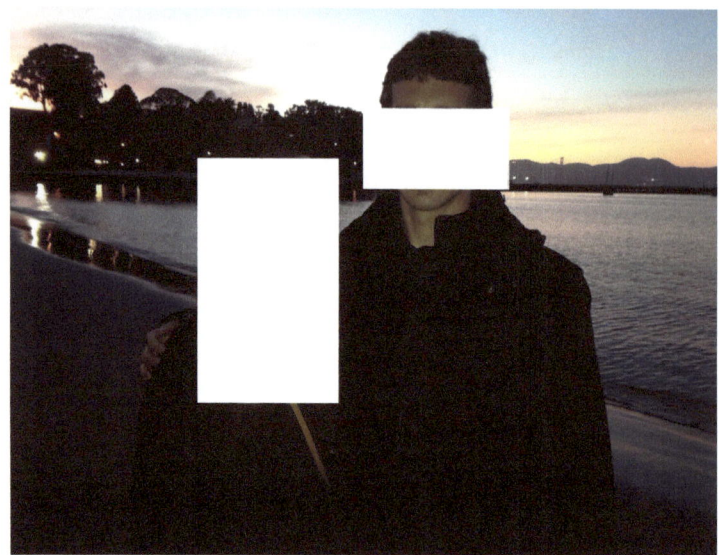

The great thing about this man and his new wife is how much they truly are open to one another and practice Tantric lovemaking. Since when he tuned his frequency to the right vibration he attracted a woman with a <u>high sex drive.</u>

Imagine if you had a lover with a high sex drive willing and eager to be with you and you didn't even have to butter her up first.

My goal for Jaime is to have many years with a woman he loves by adjusting the frequencies. We are all very different people, with very different energies-if we, learn how to work our energies there is a great chance to maintain the honeymoon passion. Sounds too good to be true, but I tell you what, the proof is RIGHT IN FRONT OF YOU. This works.

Just Imagine What the Advanced Oceans-of-Sex-Technologies™ could do for you?

I just had an "Awe Haaa!" moment.

Let me explain what I just thought.

As you know EVERYONE has sexual energies and each of those energies have a polarity.

Some naturally have more sexual energy than others.

But that is not really what I want to talk about. I'd like you to imagine for a second that you take a normal Metal bar in your hand and rub it together with another metal bar that is **already magnetized.**

Now what is about to happen is a scientific anomaly…rubbing a magnet and a metal together creates a Magnetic force that will instantly attract like objects. But you got to do the it right. You cannot switch the ends of the magnet back and forth. You must use only one side (North or South) and rub it only one way.

That non-magnetic metal pretty much <u>instantly</u> has the Magnetism transfer to it.

Pretty Cool Right? Right!

Well what if there was a REAL life **"Sexual-Energy-Magnet"** that you could "rub" and it would instantly magnetize your sexual senses?

Sounds pretty insane right? Well there IS such a thing!

The great thing about this is let's say we already have this piece of metal and it already has magnetic properties built in… And you rub it with this special magnet and your magnetism becomes even greater than a bare metal being magnetized for the first time.

Well… That is exactly where Jaime was and where you are now. Kali will help you, like Jaime, become "magnetized" with these new sexual technologies.

Lets look deeper at Jaimes story. He truely is one of my favorite success stories. Even though Jaime practically had given up on finding a nice lady… **he did one drill** and it helped allow him to act on more of his full potential.

Imagine if you could act on MORE OF YOUR full potential? How would you feel then?

Heck, imagine if you could act on half of your full potential? (According to Maslow we use less than 10% of our full potential). How would you feel then? I'll tell you, it feels "damn good"!!!

The Advanced Oceans-of-Sex-Technologies™ helps you to do things that you didn't think we're ever possible for you before.

Many people have self-improvement tools they know about that would change their life, but they, for some reason or other, are 'holding' themselves back and not grabbing their destiny by the balls. They are "stuck" and cannot move.

The Advanced Oceans-of-Sex-Technologies™ actually helped Jaime to become unstuck and just do it.

By Now, you're probably wondering How To get this Advanced Oceans-of-Sex-Training™?

Well, that might be a problem. We ONLY have a total of 130 programs in stuck and this book is a best-selling book that sells 100s of copies every day. This means 100s of people every day will know and want **Advanced Oceans-of-Sex-Training™** so if you "want one of them," call (541) 414-4277 right now or fill out the card on the next page and mail it in today.

Kali said she might up the inventory. It depends if she is going to write the 11 editions of Tantric Secrets For Men that the publisher contracted her to do.

Let me explain exactly what is **Advanced Oceans-of-Sex-Training™** it is a DVD and 7 audio program originally only sold to Kali's Inner Circle Members for $249 dollars but because you own her book and have read it which means you are interested in learning new sexual technologies, she wants you to get even more advanced technologies.

BUT $249.00 is NOT Your Price... At least NOT for today!
Your price won't even be $100.00! Or even $50.00!

We Are Just Going To Give You The Blue Print to Advanced Oceans-of-Sex-Training™ for Just $39.00

Kali will tell you the exact step-by-step process that everyone else is leaving out. And when you order this now you will find 2 bonuses.

http://www.KaliBliss.com

I am SOO EXCITED For this!!!

Just imagine the power this is going to give you. The <u>wild</u>, <u>wacky</u> and <u>wonderful</u> times you are going to have.

Enjoy my friend!

Sincerely,
Jessica Williams

P.S. When order now I am also giving you a DVD set that shows you how to use your sexual energies to influence a crowd of people. Remember the scene from Perfume, where all the character just get horny all of a sudden?

P.S.S. Remember we have limited quantities if you want one now fill out the slip below and mail it to the publishing office.

http://www.KaliBliss.com

YES! Send me "The Blue Print to Advanced Oceans-of-Sex-Training™"

My price today is just $39.00 with Shipping Included!

Make Check or Money Order Payable to Kali Bliss
Send: Check/Money Order and coupon to
Lotus Blossom Publications
33 N. Central Ave STE 204
Medford, Oregon 97501

(541) 414-4277 or call in your order!

Name:_____

Address: _____ Apt:_____ Email:_____

City:_____ State_____ Zip:_____ Phone:_____

This offer is subject to change. Please expect 2 to 3 weeks for delivery upon receipt. For any questions call Jessica the office manager at (541) 414-4277

http://www.KaliBliss.com

www.ingramcontent.com/pod-product-compliance
Lightning Source LLC
Chambersburg PA
CBHW041503280526
45792CB00004B/1118